Ketogenic Diet Cookbook

30 Keto Diet Recipes for Beginners

Easy Low Carb Plan for a Healthy Lifestyle and Quick Weight Loss

BY SANDRA WILLIAMS

TABLE OF CONTENTS

Introduction 6
    [Your Free Gift] 7
The Basic Concept 10
    What to Eat 11
    What NOT to eat 14
Breakfast 16
    Perfect Bacon 16
    Keto Spinach Feta Muffins 17
    Cinnamon Toasted Coconut Cereal 19
    Baked Avocado with Egg 21
    Buttermilk Pancakes 23
    Green Power Smoothie 25
    The Elvis (peanut butter and banana smoothie) 26
Lunch 27
    New-School Cucumber Sandwiches 27
    Ultra Veggie Soup 29
    Chicken, Bacon, Avocado Caesar Salad 30
    Simple Turkey and Swiss Wrap 31
    Broccoli Cheddar Soup 32
    Salmon Spread 33
    Greek Stuffed Burgers 34
Dinner 36
    Portobello Pizza 36
    Chicken Wings 3 Ways 38
    Slow Cooker Chili 41

    Zoodle Lasagna..43
    Taco Tuesday..45
    Classic Beef Tacos..47
    Shirataki Shrimp Stir Fry...49

Snacks..51
    Spicy Garlic Almonds...51
    Smoky, Salted Kale Chips..53
    Prosciutto e Melone..54
    Pork Rind "Popcorn"...55

Desserts..56
    Peanut Butter Mousse..56
    Berry Parfait..58
    Keto Cheesecake...59
    Mocha Bites...60
    Cinnamon Bun Bars..62
    Bonus Recipe Pumpkin Pie Squares................................64

You Can Do It..66

Conclusion...67
    Would You Like to Know More?..67

[BONUS]...68
    Preview of My Other Book, Wheat Belly Diet.......................68
    Check Out My Other Books..70

Introduction

I want to thank you and congratulate you for purchasing the book *"Ketogenic Diet Cookbook - 30 Keto Diet Recipes for Beginners, Easy Low Carb Plan for a Healthy Lifestyle and Quick Weight Loss."*

A ketogenic diet harnesses the power of high-fat, low-carb eating to rev your metabolism. These meals, snacks and desserts will keep your body burning fat as fuel all day long. Loaded with tips to help you stay on track, easy to follow recipes and grocery guidelines, this book is a MUST for any ketogenic dieter. With recipes ranging from the simple to the sophisticated, this ketogenic cookbook has meals for every taste. Whether you're looking for super easy to prepare breakfasts, or a hearty stew that cooks all day, this book has what you are looking for.

Thanks again for getting this book, I hope you'll find it useful!

PS. This is a recipe book. If you want to know what exactly is ketosis and how to go on with "low carbs" approach, check out the book **Ketogenic Diet** on Amazon here: http://bit.ly/ketodietbook

[Your Free Gift]

As a way of saying thanks for your purchase, I'm offering 2 free reports that are exclusive to my readers:

To check what are The 101 Tips That Burn Belly Fat Daily go to my page here:

=> http://projecteasylife.com/101tips <=

To see what are The 7 (Quick & Easy) Cooking Tricks To Banish Your Boring Diet go to my website here:

=> http://projecteasylife.com/7-tricks <=

© Copyright 2017 by Sandra Williams - All rights reserved.

This document is geared toward providing exact and reliable information in regards to the topic and issue covered. The publication is sold with the idea that the publisher isn't required to render accounting, officially permitted, or otherwise, qualified services. If advice is necessary, legal or professional, a practiced individual in the profession should be ordered.

From a Declaration of Principles which was accepted and approved equally by a Committee of the American Bar Association and a Committee of Publishers and Associations.

In no way is it legal to reproduce, duplicate, or transmit any part of this document in either electronic means or in printed format. Recording of this publication or any storage of this document are strictly prohibited without written permission from the publisher. All rights reserved.

The information provided herein is stated to be truthful and consistent, in that any liability, in terms of inattention or otherwise, by any usage or abuse of any policies, processes, or directions contained within is the solitary and utter responsibility of the recipient reader. Under no circumstances will any legal responsibility or blame be held against the publisher for any reparation, damages, or monetary loss due to the information herein, either directly or indirectly.

Respective authors own all copyrights not held by the publisher.

The information herein is offered for informational purposes solely, and is universal as so. The presentation of the information is without contract or any type of guarantee assurance.

The trademarks that are used are without any consent, and the publication of the trademark is without permission or backing by the trademark owner. All trademarks and brands within this book are for clarifying purposes only and are owned by the owners themselves, not affiliated with this document.

DISCLAIMER: The purpose of this book is to provide information only. The information, though believed to be entirely accurate, is NOT a substitution for medical, psychological or professional advice, diagnosis or treatment. The author recommends that you seek the advice of your physician or other qualified health care providers to present them with questions you may have regarding any medical condition. Advice from your trusted, professional medical advisor should always supersede information presented in this book.

The Basic Concept

The goal of a ketogenic diet plan is to get your body into a metabolic state called ketosis. Ketosis is a biological process in which the body burns fat cells called "ketones" instead of glucose for fuel. Establishing a state of metabolic ketosis, even for a short time frame, has many health benefits. First and foremost, adopting a ketogenic diet increases your body's ability to burn fat as fuel. The more fat you burn, the more weight you'll lose.

Any diet that limits your carbohydrate intake may be considered ketogenic. The Atkins, South Beach and Paleo diets are some famous diets you might recognize. They all work by reducing your carbohydrate/sugar consumption to allow your body to get its energy from fat (ketones) instead of sugar (glucose). They may vary in the fine details but all of them, like any ketogenic diet, involve following a higher fat, low carb food plan.

The main difference between a regular low carb diet and a ketogenic diet is the amount of carbohydrates allowed daily. While other plans might slowly increase your carb intake over time, with a ketogenic diet your daily goal should always be between 20 to 60 grams. Most of that will come from vegetables with high fiber content, which lowers the sugar impact of carbohydrates.

Most of your daily calories will come from fats. The calorie breakdown, when considered as percentages is about 70% fat, 25 % protein and 5% carbohydrates. These ratios ensure that your metabolism enters ketosis and stays there, which is the point of a ketogenic diet. It may seem impossible to lose weight while eating so much fat, but since fat kills hunger, you end up eating fewer calories without even trying.

There are many decadent foods you can eat on a ketogenic diet. Foods like bacon, heavy cream, cheeses and dark chocolate are a 'no-no' in traditional diets because of their high fat content. However, when you're are following a ketogenic eating plan, fat becomes your body's preferred energy source, making these "treats" perfectly acceptable and even encouraged. All you really need to do is base your meals around a protein source, add some vegetables and some healthy fat, and you will lose weight. If you stay in ketosis you will shed pounds. It's that simple.

What to Eat and What to Avoid On a Ketogenic Diet

On a ketogenic eating plan, the main goal is to limit your carbohydrate intake and maintain a diet on proteins and healthy fats. It may sound restrictive at first but there are tons of rich, delicious foods available to you. Below is an overview on some of the essentials.

What to Eat

Proteins

- All meat including: beef, pork, ham*, bacon*, sausages* along with venison, veal and other game meats.
- All poultry including: all cuts of chicken, Cornish hen, duck, goose, pheasant, quail, and turkey.
- All fish including shellfish.
- All eggs and fat-free eggs substitute.
- Full fat cheese and dairy: Cheddar, mozzarella, Swiss, cream cheese, cottage cheese and ricotta, plain Greek yogurt.

*Be careful with cured meats. Some use sugar and would not be allowed on a Ketogenic diet.

Oils and fats

- Butter, stick or whipped.

- Oils: canola oil, coconut oil, olive oil, safflower oil, sesame oil.

- Animal fats: Tallow (beef fat), Shortening (pork fat) or schmaltz (chicken fat).

- Mayonnaise.

- Nuts: almonds, Brazil nuts, cashews, coconut (fresh or grated, unsweetened), macadamias, hazelnuts, pecans, pine nuts, pistachios, walnuts.

- Seeds: pumpkin seeds, sunflower seeds.

Vegetables

Artichokes, arugula, asparagus, avocado, bamboo shoots, beets, bell peppers (all colors), bok choy, broccoli, broccoli rabe, Brussels sprouts, cabbage, cauliflower, celery, collard greens, cucumber, daikon, eggplant, endive, escarole, fennel, green beans (French or Italian), hearts of palm, Italian squash, jicama, leeks, lettuce (all types), mushrooms, mustard greens, okra, olives (black or green), onions, peppers, pickles, radicchio, radish, rhubarb, scallions (green onions), spaghetti squash, spinach, sprouts, summer squash, Swiss chard, tomatoes, water chestnuts, watercress, and zucchini.

Fruits

- Fruits below are your best options on a Ketogenic plan because their sugar content is low and their fiber content is very high. Still, keep portions in mind and pair them with either a fat or protein for a more nutritionally complete snack.

- Berries: blackberries, blueberries, boysenberries, currants, gooseberries, loganberries, raspberries, strawberries, cherries (sour or sweet), unsweetened cranberries.

- Melon: cantaloupe and honeydew (but not watermelon).

Beverages

- Water: tap, bottled, mineral, sparkling, flat.

- Coffee and tea (hot or iced) and espresso – zero-calories sweetener if needed (stevia.)

- Club soda and seltzer (plain or flavored, no calories).

- Diet cola, diet root beer, and other sodas (sugar-free).

- Sugar-free beverage mixes such as Kool-Aid, Crystal Light, and True Lemon.

- Milk substitutes: almond milk, coconut milk beverage (not canned coconut milk), and soy milk should be plain and sugar free.

Misc.

You may also be able to have products such as low-carb bread, chips, wraps or tortilla. Always check the label and choose product with no more than 5 carbohydrates per serving.

Alcohol is fine in small amounts. Stay away from regular beer, sweet wines and sugary mixers. Opt instead for hard alcohol (a shot). There are also several low-carb beers available. Just make sure you stay under you 60g daily carb limit.

What NOT to eat

You should avoid these foods on a ketogenic diet. While some may be a major part of other diet programs, they are loaded with sugar, which you are trying to eliminate.

- Sugar: soft drinks, fruit and vegetable juices, baked goods, candy, ice cream, etc.

- Grains: wheat, corn, barley, rice.

- Products made from flour: such as bread, pasta, pancakes, tortillas, cookies and cakes.

- Products made from corn such as cornbread, tamales, grits, polenta, and popcorn.

- High-Carb vegetables: carrots, turnips, corn, potatoes, and sweet potatoes (yams).

- Most fruit: berries and melon are the exceptions.

- Canned soups and instant noodle soups.

- Boxed, processed foods.

- Beans and legumes: kidney beans, black beans, pinto beans, lentils, and split peas.

- Milk: lactose is found in liquid milk, even in 1% and 2% varieties. The lactose is largely broken down in cheese and yogurt, which is why those foods are okay on the plan but liquid milk isn't.

- "Low-Fat" foods: fat is allowed on a Ketogenic diet. Most diet foods that reduce fat increase the sugar content.

Recipes for ketogenic eating

Now that we have gone over the guidelines and a few tips, I'll get to everyone's biggest question when starting a new healthy eating plan: "What can I eat?" The ketogenic diet is unique in that you get to eat some of the richest and most luxurious foods. No need to worry about calories or fat content. The following recipes have everything you love, from pizza and wings, to comfort classic like baked lasagna and even international fare like Asian stir fry. I even included a section for snacks and desserts (yes, DESSERT, on a low-sugar plan) that allows you to indulge your cravings, sweet or salty, creamy or crunchy, all while staying on track. Whatever you're in the mood for, there's a keto dish that can satisfy it.

Breakfast

Breakfast is the most important meal of the day. It increases your energy and starts your metabolism firing on all cylinders. Unlike some diets, they'd make you eat wheat bark every morning. Ketogenic breakfasts consist of all your favorite things like bacon, eggs, cheese and more bacon. These breakfast recipes are just what you need to put your body into fat burning mode every morning.

Perfect Bacon

Bacon may not be on your typical list of foods to eat when trying to lose weight. But ketogenic eating not only allows bacon, it lets you eat a LOT of it. Bacon is the perfect side to your breakfast, a savory topping for burgers, and a quick snack. Make a lot so you always have it on hand.

Serves 20

(43 calories per slice, 3.3g fat, 0.1g carbs, 3g protein)

Ingredients:

- 1 pound of bacon (not maple, check label for carb info)

Directions:

1. Preheat your oven to 400F.
2. Put your slices of bacon into one even layer on a baking sheet. The cook time is the same for 1 slice or dozen, so make a sizable batch to get the most out of your time.
3. Place tray in the oven, cook 15 minutes for chewy bacon and up to 20 for crisp bacon.
4. Allow bacon to cool and continue to crisp on pan before serving or storing.

Keto Spinach Feta Muffins

Eggs are a staple of the ketogenic diet. But sometimes mornings can be hectic and you simply don't have time to cook. Whip up a batch of these make-ahead omelet muffins. They are the perfect grab-and-go breakfast. And since each serving is cooked in its own muffin cup, you can make 12 different flavors all at once, or a dozen of your favorite.

Serves 6

(220 calories per muffin, 16g fat, 3g carbs, 12g protein)

Ingredients:

- 6 eggs
- 3 slices bacon, cooked
- 2 c. raw spinach
- 1 c. crumbled feta cheese
- ½ c. cheddar cheese
- Salt and pepper to taste

Directions:

1. Preheat oven to 350F. Rinse the spinach under cold water, drain and place in a microwave safe bowl. Microwave the spinach on high for 1 minute. (there will be enough moisture left on the rinsed leaves to cook the spinach). Set aside to cool.

2. If you happen to have leftover cooked bacon, you could use that. But who am I kidding, nobody has leftover cooked

bacon. You'll have to chop this bacon up and fry it until it's how you like it. Set aside to cool.

3. In a medium mixing bowl, whisk the eggs together until frothy. Add in the crumbled feta cheese and the grated cheddar cheese. Once the spinach and bacon are cooled enough, add them to the bowl and mix until combined.

4. Divide the mixture evenly among the 6 muffin cups. Bake for 30-35 minutes until muffins are firm.

Cinnamon Toasted Coconut Cereal

You should know by now that grains and cereals are not allowed on a ketogenic eating plan. But sometimes a big bowl of cereal is exactly what you are craving. Opt instead for this low-carb alternative that packs the same crunch but without undermining your weight loss goals.

Serves 4

(495 calories per serving, 59g fat, 16.72g carbs, 8.85g fiber, 7.87g net carbs, 2.57g protein)

Ingredients:

- 7 oz. unsweetened Coconut Flakes (about 3 1/2 cups)
- 2 T. butter or ghee
- 2 T. cinnamon
- ¼ c. granular sweetener (Also can use coconut sugar or swerve)

Directions:

1. Preheat your oven to 350F degrees.
2. Place the coconut flakes in a large bowl.
3. In a saucepan, over medium heat, combine the butter, cinnamon, and sweetener and heat until thoroughly incorporated.
4. Pour the sauce over the coconut and stir to coat
5. Spread the coconut onto a rimmed baking sheet.

6. Bake for 5-8 minutes, stirring and flipping the coconut every few minutes so they don't burn.

7. Allow to cool and serve with almond or coconut milk.

Notes:

Net Carb Count*: 7.87 g net carbs (per serving - serves 4. Add the carbs for the sweetener you use.)

Total Carb Count: 16.72 g total carbs (per serving - serves 4. Add the carbs for the sweetener you use.)

*Note net carb count = Total carbs – fiber. Carb counts are estimated based on the products. Check nutrition labels for accurate carb counts and gluten information.

Baked Avocado with Egg

This breakfast is exactly what the ketogenic diet is about. A blend of health fat and protein. While bacon and eggs make for a delicious way to start the day, even that can be boring after a while. Mix up your a.m. basics with rich and satisfying egg dish. This is the basic recipe, but feel free to add fresh herbs or a sprinkling of cheese to customize it to your taste.

Serves 4

(224 calories per serving, 19g fat, 7g fiber, 9g net carbs, 8g protein)

Ingredients:

- 2 ripe avocados
- 4 fresh eggs
- Pinch of salt and pepper

Directions:

1. Place the rack in the center of the oven and preheat to 425F degrees.
2. Slice the avocados in half vertically, and remove the pit. Scoop out additional flesh, about 1 ½ to 2 tablespoons worth, from the center of the avocado. You want enough room for the eggs to fill the center without overflowing.
3. Place the avocados in a small baking dish. Use the smallest dish that will fit them.
4. You don't want them to have a ton of room to wiggle or slide around.

5. Separate one egg at a time. Place the yolk in the avocado and then fill up the remaining space with the white. Discard any unused white or save for another recipe.

6. Place in the tray in the oven and bake for 15 - 20 minutes. Cooking times vary depending on the size of the eggs and avocados. Cook just until the whites are set but the yolk remains runny.

7. Remove from oven, then season with pepper. Garnish however you choose.

Buttermilk Pancakes

A classic is a classic for a reason. Giving up grains doesn't mean never again having golden, fluffy delicious pancakes for breakfast. That would just be plain cruel. With a few low-carb substitutions, these ketogenic pancakes put short stacks (and tall ones too) back on the menu.

Serving sizes can vary depending on preference

(86 calories per 4" pancake, 3.53g fat, 10.91g carbs, 7g fiber, 7.87g net carbs, 2.58g protein)

Ingredients:

- 6 eggs, separated (you need 2 yolks and 6 whites)
- 1/2 c. buttermilk
- 1 tsp. vanilla extract
- 1 T. vanilla protein powder
- 1/4 c. finely milled coconut flour
- 1 tsp. baking powder
- 1 packet stevia
- Butter flavored cooking spray

Directions:

1. Using a hand mixer with a whisk attachment, beat two egg whites with a pinch of salt until soft peaks form. Set aside.
2. In a separate bowl, mix the buttermilk, egg yolks, remaining egg whites, and vanilla extract together very well.

3. In a separate bowl, whisk the coconut flour, protein powder, and baking powder.

4. Add the dry ingredients to the wet and mix until combined.

5. Fold the whipped egg whites into the batter. Be careful not to over mix or you will deflate the egg whites and they will become runny.

6. Preheat a nonstick skillet over medium-low heat.

7. Spray the pan liberally with cooking spray.

8. Pour 1/4 cup of batter into the skillet.

9. Cook until small bubbles begin to form and are visible on top.

10. Flip the pancake, just once, and cook until the other side is golden brown.

Green Power Smoothie

Potent and portable, green smoothies are a big trend in food right now. This ketogenic green smoothie packs a one-two punch of metabolism boosting healthy fat and nutrient rich veggies.

Serves 1

(460 calories per serving, 43.3g fat, 13g carbs, 6.5g protein)

Ingredients:

- ¼ avocado
- 2 c. baby spinach, torn
- 1 Persian cucumber, diced
- ½ c. full-fat coconut cream
- 1 T., 1 tsp. Tahini
- 2 tsp. coconut oil
- 1 tsp. alfalfa powder greens supplement
- Ice
- 1½ - 2 c. water

Directions:

1. Add all ingredients to a blender, adding only a small amount of water at the start.
2. Blend until smooth, adding water until you reach your desired consistency.

The Elvis (peanut butter and banana smoothie)

A great a.m. treat to boost your energy and curb your sweet tooth, all while staying on track.

Serves 1

(374 calories per serving, 9g fat, 36g carbs, 5g fiber, 31g net carbs, 39g protein)

Ingredients:

- 1 c. unsweetened almond milk
- ¼ c., 1 T. whipped cream
- 1 scoop sugar-free chocolate protein powder
- 1 tsp. low-sugar peanut butter
- 1 tsp. unsweetened cocoa powder
- 1 tsp. banana extract
- ½ c. coffee, room temperature
- ½ tsp. xanthan gum (optional)

Directions:

1. Add all ingredients to a blender and mix until well combined. Add xanthan gum to achieve a thicker texture.

Lunch

For some people, a ketogenic breakfast satisfies their hunger so much that they skip lunch altogether. For others, 3 full meals are doable. Listen to your body and eat when you're hungry. Each person is different. For lunch, the key thing is keeping it quick and easy. For this we are going to focus on the 3S's – Soups, Salads and Sandwiches. These ketogenic lunches are great because they're customizable. Here are some essential recipes, but feel free to substitute whichever meats, veggies and cheeses you prefer.

New-School Cucumber Sandwiches

Cucumber sandwiches are usually seen at English tea services and luncheons. Here we give it a ketogenic spin, replacing slices of lightly toasted white bread with cucumber itself. We kept the classic cream cheese flavor (with a twist) and added some lean meat for a protein boost.

Serves 1

(391 calories per serving, 27.9g fat, 9.5g carbs, 23.8g protein)

Ingredients:

- 1 Cucumber
- 1 T. spreadable cheese such as Boursin or Rondele
- 4 thin slices deli-style roast beef

Directions:

1. Using a vegetable peeler, carefully remove the skin of the cucumber.

2. Cut the cucumber in half length-wise (like a hamburger bun) and use a teaspoon to scoop out the seeds and create an even edge all the way around the cucumber.
3. Fill one side with a spreadable cheese.
4. Fold deli meat and tuck it into the other half of the cucumber.
5. Stack the two halves back on top of each other and cut again, the same way you would cut a sandwich in half.

Note: Boursin and roast beef is a great combination. Also, try turkey with veggie cream cheese or ham with white cheddar.

Ultra Veggie Soup

Veggies are your friends. They help fill you up, help regulate blood sugar and aid in digestion. This vegetarian vegetable soup is full of fiber and will keep you full throughout your day. You can always switch out any veggie you dislike or add more of your favorites. Just make sure you are choosing low carb veggies. You can also bulk it up with diced chicken or turkey breast for a heartier meal.

Serves 4

(95 calories per serving, 7.6g fat, 6.7g carbs, 4.2g fiber, 2.5g net carbs, 2.1g protein)

Ingredients:

- 2 c. spinach leaves
- 1 avocado
- 1/2 c. English cucumber
- 1 green onion
- 1/2 c. red bell pepper
- 1/4 c. gluten-free vegetable broth
- 1 garlic clove
- 1 T. braggs soy seasoning
- 1 T. lemon juice
- pinch chili powder (optional)
- freshly ground pepper, to taste

Directions:

1. Throw all ingredients in the blender and blend until smooth.

Chicken, Bacon, Avocado Caesar Salad

Without a tasty dressing, a salad is just a pile of bland veggies. Most bottled varieties are full of starchy fillers, high fructose corn syrup and other foods bad for your metabolism. This rich and thick Caesar dressing is a cinch to make and can also be a great marinade for chicken or fish.

Serves 2

(337 calories per serving, 27g fat, 3g carbs, 19g protein)

Ingredients:

- 1 ripe avocado, sliced
- 1 chicken breast (grilled/precooked)
- 1 c. crumbled bacon
- 3 T. Marie's Creamy Caesar dressing

Directions:

1. Slice avocado in half, twist, and discard pit. Slice in half, then easily remove the shell. Slice into about 1" slices.
2. Slice your pre-cooked/grilled chicken breast into slices.
3. Between two bowls, combine avocado slices, chicken breast, and crumbled bacon.
4. Top with a few dollops of creamy Caesar dressing and lightly toss (careful not to smoosh the avocado).
5. Enjoy!

Simple Turkey and Swiss Wrap

Serves 1

(194 calories per serving, 6.32g fat, 16.5g carbs, 4.49g protein)

Ingredients:
- 2 turkey slices
- 1 wedge spreadable Swiss cheese (such as Laughing Cow)
- 1/2 c. salad greens such as baby spinach or kale
- 1 T. stone ground mustard
- 1 low-carb 6" sandwich wrap

Directions:
1. Smear one side of wrap with Swiss cheese spread.
2. Cover the lower half of the wrap with veggies.
3. Layer the turkey on top of that and finish with spicy mustard.
4. Fold in the sides of the wrap and then roll to close.
5. Makes one serving.

Broccoli Cheddar Soup

Serves 8

(291 calories per serving, 25g fat, 5g carbs, 13g protein)

Ingredients:

- 4 minced garlic cloves
- 3 ½ c. low sodium chicken broth (or vegetable broth)
- 4 c. broccoli (cut into florets)
- 1 c. heavy cream (whipping cream)
- 3 c. shredded cheddar cheese

Directions:

1. In a large pot over medium heat, sautée garlic for one minute, over fragrant.
2. Add the chicken broth, heavy cream, and chopped broccoli. Increase heat to bring to a boil, then reduce heat and simmer for 15-20 minutes, until broccoli is tender.
3. Add the shredded cheese gradually, stirring consistently, and continue to stir until melted. (Add ½ cup, simmer and stir until it melts fully, then repeat ½ cup at a time until all the cheese is used up.) Remove from heat immediately once all the cheese melts.

Salmon Spread

This simple and flavorful spread is a cinch to make and has seemingly endless uses. Serve on a bed of salad greens, as a dip for veggies or make a sandwich with low-carb bread or wraps.

Serves 8

(254.5 calories per serving, 26.18g fat, 4.61g carbs, 4.98g protein)

Ingredients:

- 1 c. full-fat cream cheese
- ⅔ c. organic butter
- 1 package (3.5oz) boneless smoked salmon
- 1 T. lemon juice
- 1 T. dried dill
- Salt and Pepper for taste

Directions:

1. In a food processor, combine cream cheese, butter and smoked salmon.
2. Add the lemon juice and dill. Pulse a few times until mixture is smooth and uniform. Add salt and pepper if desired.
3. Keep refrigerated until ready to serve. Store in an air tight container.

Greek Stuffed Burgers

Serves 6

(506.3 calories per serving, 21.2g fat, 35.9g carbs, 38.5g protein)

Ingredients:

- 2 lbs. 90% lean ground beef
- ½ c. feta cheese, crumbled
- ½ c. tomatoes, chopped
- 2 T. red onions, chopped
- 2 T. ripe olives, chopped
- 1 T. olive oil
- ¼ tsp. dried oregano
- ½ tsp. salt
- ¼ tsp. pepper
- 6 whole gyro style pita bread (6 inches)
- 6 lettuce leaves
- 6 slices tomatoes
- 1 small seedless cucumber, sliced
- ⅓ c. cucumber ranch salad dressing

Directions:

1. Shape beef evenly into 12 patties.
2. In a small bowl, combine the feta cheese, chopped tomato, onion, olives, oil and oregano.

3. Top six of the patties with the cheese mixture and then cover with remaining patties and firmly press edges to seal. Sprinkle with salt and pepper for seasoning.
4. Grill patties, covered over medium hot heat for 6-8 minutes on each side or until a meat thermometer reads 160F and juices are clear.
5. Serve each burger on a pita with lettuce, sliced tomato, cucumber and cucumber ranch dressing.

Dinner

It's the end of the day. You've stayed on track all day. Don't derail your dedication by giving in to tempting pastas, pizza and tacos. Instead have these keto-friendly versions of your favorites.

Portobello Pizza

Serves 3

(276 calories per serving, 21g fat, 6g carbs 19g protein)

Ingredients:

- 3 Portobello Mushrooms
- Drizzle of Olive Oil
- 1 T. pizza seasoning
- 3 tomato slices
- 9 spinach leaves
- 1.5 oz. mozzarella
- 1.5 oz. Monterey Jack
- 1.5 oz. cheddar cheese
- 12 pepperoni slices

Directions:

1. Preheat Convection Oven to 450F.
2. Wash and destem the Portobello Mushrooms.

3. Place the mushrooms cap side down on a foil lined sheet and drizzle with olive oil.
4. Sprinkle with pizza seasoning.
5. Layer spinach, tomato, cheese and another round of seasoning.
6. Cook in the convection oven until cheese has melted or around 6 minutes.
7. Add the pepperoni and cook until the pepperoni is crispy.

Chicken Wings 3 Ways

Perfect for game day, these wings are a great time saver because you only need to cook once to get 3 different and distinct wings. The same spice mix goes on the wings before they bake, and the product depends on which tasty sauce you lather it in: spicy buffalo, garlicky parmesan or sweet teriyaki.

Garlic Parmesan Chicken Wings

Serves 12

(270.7 calories per serving, 20.7g fat, 0.5g carbs, 19.7g protein)

Ingredients:

- ¼ c. butter, melted
- 1 tsp. garlic powder
- ½ tsp. onion salt
- ¼ tsp. black pepper, freshly ground
- ½ c. parmesan cheese, grated
- 12 chicken wings, nude, baked (or fried per your desire)

Directions:

1. In a small glass bowl, melt butter in microwave.
2. Whisk into butter the garlic powder, onion salt and pepper.
3. Arrange hot, fresh-baked nude wings on a serving platter and drizzle with butter mixture.
4. Top with parmesan cheese and serve immediately.

Buffalo Chicken Wings

Serves 12

(228.6 calories per serving, 16.1g fat, 2.1g carbs, 17.6g protein)

Ingredients:

- Oil, for frying
- 12 chicken wings
- ¼ c. all-purpose flour
- 1 tsp. garlic salt
- ½ tsp. seasoning salt
- buffalo sauce
- 1 T. butter, melted
- 1 T. white vinegar
- ½ tsp. garlic, crushed
- ¼ tsp. onion powder
- 2 -3 tsp. red pepper sauce (to taste)
- ¼ tsp. salt

Directions:
1. Heat oil in fryer.
2. Cut each chicken wing at joints to make 3 pieces and discard the tip.
3. Combine the flour garlic and seasoning salt in gallon size zip lock bag.
4. Place chicken in bag and shack until it's all well coated.
5. Fry in fryer until done.

6. Remove chicken to a paper towel lined dish and drain.
7. Meanwhile, mix the buffalo ingredients into a bowl.
8. Add chicken and toss until evenly coated with buffalo mixture.

Teriyaki Chicken Wings

Serves 12

(261 calories per serving, 11.6g fat, 9.9g carbs, 28.1g protein)

Ingredients:
- Oil, for frying
- 12 chicken wings
- 1/3 c. sugar
- ¼ c. brown sugar
- 1 tsp. garlic powder
- 1 tsp. ground ginger
- ½ c. soy sauce
- 1/3 c. water
- 2 T. pineapple juice

Directions:
1. Warm oil over medium heat
2. Marinade 12 chicken wings
3. Fry in fryer until done.

Slow Cooker Chili

A hearty bowl of warm chili is perfect all year round. From cold winter's nights, barbeques and tail gates, this no-bean chili recipe has you covered. Cooking it on low for several hours lets the flavors meld and develop that rich, satisfying taste that you want from chili. After browning the meat, mix everything together and wait. Your patience will be rewarded.

One cup per serving

(187 calories per serving, 5g fat, 4.7g carbs, 16g protein)

Ingredients:

- 2 1/2 lbs. ground beef
- 1 medium red onion, chopped and divided
- ¼ c. minced garlic
- 3 large ribs of celery, diced
- ¼ c. pickled jalapeno slices
- 6 oz. can tomato paste
- 14.5 oz. canned tomatoes and green chilies
- 14.5 oz. canned stewed tomatoes with Mexican seasoning
- 2 T. Worcestershire sauce
- ¼ c. chili powder
- 2 T. cumin, mounded
- 2 tsp. sea salt
- 1/2 tsp. cayenne
- 1 tsp. garlic powder

- 1 tsp. onion powder
- 1 tsp. oregano
- 1 tsp. black pepper
- 1 bay leaf

Directions:

1. Heat slower cooker on low setting.
2. In a larger skillet over medium-high heat, add ground beef, half of the onions, two tablespoons minced garlic, salt and pepper. Once beef is browned, drained excess grease from pan.
3. Transfer ground beef mixture to slow cooker. Add remaining onions, garlic, celery, jalapenos, tomato paste, tomatoes and chilies (with liquid), stewed tomatoes (with liquid), Worcestershire sauce, chili powder, salt, cayenne powder, garlic powder, onion powder, oregano, black pepper and bay leaf.
4. Stir until ingredients are well combined. Cook on low 6-8 hours.

Zoodle Lasagna

What is a Zoodle? A zucchini noodle. Replacing starchy lasagna noodles with thinly sliced zucchini allows this ketogenic classic deliver all the cheesy goodness of a traditional lasagna.

Serves 4

(281calories per serving, 18.1g fat, 15.5g carbs, 16.1g protein)

Ingredients:

- 4 zucchinis, sliced 1/4" thick
- 1 ½ c. tomato sauce
- 1 c. grated Parmigiano Reggiano cheese
- 2/3 c. shredded mozzarella cheese
- 1 ½ c. béchamel sauce

Directions:

1. Preheat oven to 375F.
2. Cut zucchini lengthwise into 1/4-inch thick slices with a knife or mandolin.
3. Pour 2 tablespoons tomato sauce on the bottom of a 9x13-inch baking dish. Arrange zucchini slices in a single layer, slightly overlapping, over tomato sauce.
4. Top with a thin layer of mozzarella, 1/3 of the bechamel (see Editor's Note), 1/3 of remaining tomato sauce, 1/3 of the Parmigiano Reggiano cheese, and 1/3 of the basil.

Repeat layers, topping with bechamel and Parmigiano Reggiano cheese.
5. Bake in the preheated oven until sauce is bubbly and the top is golden brown, about 35 minutes. Allow to set until remaining liquid is absorbed, about 10 minutes.

Taco Tuesday

Perfect tacos need two main things, a great tasty taco shell and a super flavorful seasoning mix. Here, I have recipes for both, as well as a simple easy way to tie it all together.

No-carb Taco Shell

Serves 1

(151.6 calories per serving, 12.5g fat, 0.5g carbs, 9.4g protein)

Ingredients:

- 1/3 cup cheddar cheese

Directions:

1. Place 1/3 cup of cheese in thin layer on parchment paper.
2. Microwave on high for one minute, or until cheese is bubbly.
3. While the cheese is still flexible with parchment paper still attached, bend the cheese over a round object to give it a taco shell shape.
4. The smaller in diameter the object is, the closer to a normal taco shell shape you will have.
5. Let the cheese cool while around the object.
6. When it has cooled, peel it from the parchment paper.

Perfecto Taco Seasoning

The key to a great ground beef taco is in the spice mix. Unfortunately, the pre-mixed seasoning blends from the market are usually loaded with sugar. Use this simple blend to eliminate carbs while still getting full flavor. You'll save money and you won't have to give up tacos. The spice mix easily doubles. It's great for chili, Mexican stews and anything you want to have that extra little kick.

Ingredients:

- 1 T. chili powder
- ½ tsp. onion powder
- ½ tsp. garlic powder
- ½ tsp. Mexican oregano
- 1½ tsp. cumin
- 1 tsp. salt
- 1 tsp. black pepper
- For Spicy add: 1 pinch cayenne pepper
- For Extra spicy also add: 1 pinch red pepper flakes

Directions:

1. Mix all spices together.
2. Store in an airtight container until ready to use.

Classic Beef Tacos

Serves 8

(107 calories per serving, 7g fat, 0.8g carbs, 9.7g protein)

Ingredients:

- 1 lb. ground beef
- ¼ tsp. dried oregano
- ¼ tsp. dried minced garlic
- ¼ tsp. cayenne pepper (optional)
- ½ tsp. red pepper flakes
- ½ tsp. ground cumin
- ½ tsp. cornstarch
- 1 tsp. chili powder
- 1 tsp. salt
- 2 tsp. dried minced onion

Directions:

1. Mix minced onion, salt, chili pepper, cornstarch, cumin, red pepper flakes, cayenne pepper, dried minced garlic, and oregano in a bowl.

2. Heat a large skillet over medium-high heat. Crumble ground beef into the hot skillet. Cook and stir until beef is completely brown, 7-10 min. Drain and discard any excess grease.

3. Return ground beef to heat. Pour seasoning mixture and water over the beef; stir to combine. Bring to a simmer and cook until moisture absorbs into the meat, about 5 minutes.

*If you prefer, you can substitute low carb tortillas and taco shells from the market, though I recommend the No-carb Shell from this book. You can also skip the shell altogether and eat this as a salad. Just double up on the lettuce.

Shirataki Shrimp Stir Fry

Shirataki is a blessing for anyone on a ketogenic diet. Made from yams these noodles have NO carbs. Great for any dish that requires thin noodles. Such as this Thai-inspired stir fry dish.

Serves 2

(237 calories, 13.15g fat, 7.6g carbs, 17.8g protein)

Ingredients:

- 24 medium shrimp, peeled and deveined
- 2 8-oz. packages of tofu *shirataki* noodles (Konjac noodles)
- 1½ T. coconut oil
- 2 oz. onion, slivered into thin strips
- 2 oz. red bell pepper, slivered into thin strips
- 1 very large jalapeno, seeded and slivered into thin strips
- 1 clove garlic, minced
- ¼ tsp. ginger root, peeled and minced
- 1 T. sherry or white wine (omit if on Induction)
- 1 T. low-sodium soy sauce
- Pinch sesame seed seasoning (or toasted sesame seeds)
- 1 c. chicken broth (homemade) or 1 cube in 1 c. water
- 1/8 tsp. xanthan gum

Directions:

1. Open bags of noodles and rinse them for 3-4 minutes under hot water to remove the fishy odor. Drain on paper

toweling. The shrimp topping will eliminate any remaining odor on the noodles after rinsing. Set aside.

2. Prepare all the vegetables and have them at the ready by the stove. Crumble the bouillon cube into the hot water. Add soy sauce, garlic and ginger.

3. Heat coconut oil in a non-stick wok or skillet. Stir-fry the onion, red pepper and jalapeno until it begins to get tender. Add shrimp and sautee until they're curling and opaque.

4. Pour chicken bouillon mixture into pan and sautee 1-2 minutes. Sprinkle xanthan gum over top of mixture and stir/sautee 1-2 minutes or until it begins to slightly thicken the sauce and the liquid is adhering to the shrimp and veggies. Turn fire off.

5. Fill half the noodles on each of two dinner plates and dip half the shrimp mixture up over the noodles. Serve with a lovely green salad.

Snacks

Because fat and protein curb your appetite on fewer calories, people who follow a ketogenic diet tend not to snack much. They often feel perfectly satisfied with the basic 3 meals per day. However, if you're hungry in between meals, here are a few quick snacks that will satisfy your cravings and keep you on track.

Spicy Garlic Almonds

Serves 8 (1/4 c.)

(225 calories per serving, 19g fat, 7g carbs, 7g protein)

Ingredients:

- 2 c. whole unsalted almonds
- 1tsp. ground cumin
- ¼ tsp. garlic powder
- ¼ tsp. cayenne powder
- ½ tsp. salt
- 2 tsp. olive oil
- ¼ tsp. hot pepper sauce

Directions:

1. Toast the almonds in a dry skillet over a medium heat, stirring frequently, until fragrant, about 3 minutes. Transfer the almonds to a bowl.

2. In a small bowl, stir together the cumin, garlic, cayenne pepper and salt.

3. Heat the oil in the skillet over medium heat. Stir the spices into the oil and cook, stirring until warm, about 30 seconds. Add the almonds and cook, stirring frequently, until the nuts are warm and the spices are evenly distributed. Add the hot pepper sauce and stir to distribute.

4. Remove the almonds from the pan and allow them to cool before serving.

Smoky, Salted Kale Chips

The secret to a perfectly crisp kale chip is not overcrowding the pan. Because of this, only half a bunch of kale is used per sheet pan. You can easily double up this recipe, either by repeating the process or by cooking two pans side by side in the oven.

Serves 8 (1 cup per serving)

(60 calories per serving, 4g fat, 6g carbs, 2g protein)

Ingredients:

- 1 bunch kale, about 8 c.
- 1 T. olive oil
- 1 tsp. smoked paprika
- 1/4 tsp. salt

Directions:

1. Remove the center ribs and stems from 1 bunch kale; tear the leaves into 3-4-inch pieces. Toss with 1 tablespoon olive oil, 1 teaspoon smoked paprika and 1/4 teaspoon salt.

2. Spread on 2 baking sheets coated with cooking spray. Bake at 350F until browned around the edges and crisp, 12-15 minutes.

Prosciutto e Melone

This classic Italian start is a perfect ketogenic snack. The key to getting the best taste out of such basic ingredients is by purchasing high quality ham and fresh fruits. Mixing sweet melon and salty prosciutto makes this quick snack super simple and tasty.

Serves 4

(99 calories per serving, 4.8g fat, 11.3g carbs, 3.9g protein)

Ingredients:

- 1 cantaloupe, seeded and cut into 8 wedges
- 8 thin slices prosciutto

Directions:

1. Remove the rind and seeds from the cantaloupe. Wrap each wedge with a slice of prosciutto. Serve at room temperature.

Pork Rind "Popcorn"

Popcorn isn't a ketogenic snack, but it's a snack that people love. Try this replacement, using pork rinds, to get that salty, butter taste we all love.

Serves 1

(174 calories per serving, 10.02g fat, 0g carb, 19.62g protein)

Ingredients:

- 3 oz. plain pork rinds bag
- 1 T. Italian seasoning
- 2 tsp. Parmesan cheese
- 1 tsp. salt (popcorn salt if available)
- Dash pepper
- 2 T. butter

Directions:

1. Spread the pork rinds out in a large baking dish.
2. In a small bowl, stir together the Parmesan, Italian seasoning salt and pepper.
3. Place the butter in a microwave safe dish and microwave at 50% power until melted (about 1 minute).
4. Drizzle melted butter over the pork rinds while shaking the dish to evenly distribute the butter on all sides of the rinds.
5. Sprinkle with the seasoning mixture.
6. Toss to coat.

Desserts

Sweet tooth? These desserts will trick you into thinking you're indulging. Fruity, rich, light, even peanut buttery. The following desserts are sure to satisfy.

Peanut Butter Mousse

Serves 4-6 (serving size 1/3c.)

(247 calories per serving, 22g fat, 8.8g carbs, 3.8g protein)

Ingredients:

- 1 can full fat unsweetened coconut milk
- 3-4 T. salted, natural creamy peanut butter
- 2-3 T. honey

Directions:

1. Chill your coconut milk overnight. In the morning, without shaking or tipping, remove the lid and scoop out the solid cream from the top into a chilled bowl.
2. Using a mixer, beat until creamed together, light and fluffy - about 45 seconds.
3. Add peanut butter, starting with 2 T. and adding from there to desired taste.
4. Add sweetener of choice to desired sweetness, observing that the more liquid you add the less firm the mousse will be.

5. Either use immediately as a spreadable frosting, or chill for several hours to let it set and firm up as a mousse.
6. Eat as a mousse topped with plain coconut whipped cream, bananas or chocolate sauce. Alternatively, use as a dip for fruit/baked goods. If using as a frosting, don't frost your muffins, cookies and cakes, etc., until just before serving as it needs to be chilled right up until serving.
7. Reserve leftovers in a covered container in the fridge. Will keep for up to 1 week.

Berry Parfait

Serves 6

(185 calories per serving, 7.2g fat, 24g carbs, 3.1g protein)

Ingredients:

- 1/3 c. strawberries
- 1/3 c. blueberries
- ½ c. raspberries
- ½ c. blackberries
- 1 pint vanilla frozen yogurt
- 1 (8 oz.) container frozen whipped topping, thawed

Directions:

1. In a blender, combine blueberries, strawberries and whipped topping. Blend until smooth. Transfer to a mixing bowl and fold in raspberries and blackberries. Layer the berry mixture with the frozen yogurt in 6 dessert glasses, finishing with a berry layer. Serve at once.

2. Leftover cream can be stored in the fridge and whipped again for reuse. Another great tip is to make the parfait using frozen berries. Build the dish in the evening and put it in the fridge overnight. In the morning, you can have a luscious sweet treat to break up your routine.

Keto Cheesecake

The king of desserts, this fluffy and creamy slice of heaven tastes like the original and is completely sugar-free. Be sure to serve at your next family dinner event, top it with fresh berries of sugar-free chocolate ganache to exceed the limit.

Serves 10

(278 calories per serving, 26.7g fat, 3.31g carbs, 3.31g protein)

Ingredients:

- 3 8 oz. packages of cream cheese, room temperature
- 1 c. stevia
- 1 tsp. vanilla extract
- 1/3 c. sour cream
- 4 eggs

Directions:

1. Preheat oven to 350F. Beat cream cheese until fluffy, about 3 minutes. Combine with sweetener, sour cream and vanilla extract, mixing for about 3 minutes.
2. Gently add eggs one at a time, beating until thick and creamy, about one minute after each egg.
3. Lightly grease the sides of a 9" springform pan and put it on a baking sheet. Pour in the filling. Bake for 50-55 minutes or until puffy and lightly brown around the edges.
4. Let cool for about 1-2 hours on wire rack. Cover, refrigerate for at least four hours.

Mocha Bites

With a classic mix of coffee, chocolate, and a texture that's part cheesecake and part ice cream, these mocha bites are everything your sweet tooth is after.

Serves 8

(98 calories per serving, 8.9g fat, 1.25g carbs, 1.1g protein)

Ingredients:

- 1 8 oz. cream cheese, softened
- ¼ c. organic butter
- 2 T. coconut oil
- 2 T. unsweetened cocoa powder
- ¼ c. stevia for baking
- 10-15 drops liquid stevia
- ½ cup coffee, room temperature

Directions:

1. Place the softened cream cheese, coconut oil, cocoa powder and both types of stevia into a blender and pulse until well combined.
2. Pour in the coffee and pulse again until smooth.
3. *Pour into an ice-cream maker and process for 30-60 minutes, depending on the maker you use.
4. Spoon the ice-cream base into an air-tight container.
5. Place into the freezer for 2-3 hours or until firm.

*You can skip using the ice cream maker if you don't have one. Simply pour the mix right into a freezer safe container. The flavor will be the same but the texture won't be as smooth.

Cinnamon Bun Bars

Missing your baked goods on keto? Get your gooey cinnamon bun fix with these frozen keto bars that mimic those starchy, sugary treats you've been craving.

Serves 8

(180 calories per serving, 18.1g fat, 2.7g carbs, 2.9g protein)

Ingredients:

Bottom layer

- 1 c. coconut cream
- ¼ tsp. cinnamon

Middle layer

- 2 T. extra virgin coconut oil
- 2 T. almond butter

Top layer

- 2 T. almond butter
- 1 tsp. cinnamon

Directions:

1. Line a square (9x9) cake pan with parchment paper.
2. Mix the coconut cream and cinnamon (bottom layer). Spread evenly into cake pan.
3. In a bowl, whisk together the coconut oil and almond butter (middle layer). Spread evenly on top of the creamed coconut layer and place in the freezer for 10 minutes.

4. Combine almond butter and cinnamon. Drizzle this final icing over the bars and freeze another 5 minutes.

5. Cut into rectangular bars.

6. Keep chilled until ready to serve.

Bonus Recipe Pumpkin Pie Squares

Serves 4

(300 calories per serving, 32.38g fat, 1.43g carbs, 1.4g protein)

Ingredients:

- ½ c. organic butter
- ½ c. pureed pumpkin (do NOT use pumpkin pie filling, it's loaded with sugar)
- ½ c. mascarpone cheese
- ¼ c. stevia
- 1 tsp. ground cinnamon
- ½ tsp. pumpkin spice
- Pinch salt
- 2 tsp. vanilla extract

Directions:

1. Melt butter over medium heat, stirring often to prevent burning.
2. Add pureed pumpkin and whisk.
3. Add cream cheese, sweetener, cinnamon and pie spice. Whisk until smooth.
4. Add vanilla extract. Mix completely and remove from heat.
5. Line a square cake pan (9X9) with parchment paper and pour mixture.

6. Place into the freezer for at least 24 hours. When ready to slice, cut into 9 square like a tic-tac-toe pattern.

7. Store in an air-tight container in the freezer until ready to serve.

You Can Do It

You now have all the tools you need to be successful on a ketogenic eating plan. You know which foods to eat and avoid. You have some great dishes to start your day with, quick and simple lunches and hearty dinners. You have some snacks to curb cravings and desserts to satisfy your sweet tooth. You don't have to concern yourself with calories, fat or points. If you stay under your daily carb limit, you'll lose a significant amount of weight. Here are some final tips for getting the most out of your new way of eating.

Tip for success: Get a carb counting book and small notebook. Studies show that people who track what they eat while dieting lose 3 times more weight than those who don't. Having a carb total book will help you stay within your daily range. Writing it down helps tracking become a habit.

Tip for success: Stay hydrated. Drinking plenty of fluids helps you in so many ways. It's key in helping your body flush out fat and toxins, it revs your metabolism and helps you feel fuller throughout the day. Water should be your "go to" beverage. Make sure you are drinking plenty of water (6-8 glasses daily). Try adding a twist of lemon or lime for zest.

Tip for Success: To get off to a great start, clear your fridge and pantry of all foods and ingredients that aren't keto-friendly. Don't rely solely on willpower. If it isn't in the house, you won't be tempted. Get rid of sugary treats like candies, ice cream, and soda as well are carbohydrate laden items like bread, pasta, and cereal.

Congratulations on starting a ketogenic plan. Enjoy making (and most importantly eating) these tasty meals.

Conclusion

Thanks for reading my book to the end! ☺

Now I would like to ask for a *small* favor. I am self-published author, and if you liked my book, a review on Amazon would be a great help for me. This feedback will let me continue to write the kind of books that will help people and will let me improve.

Go to http://bit.ly/ketocookreview if you'd like to leave a review, and thanks in advance for any kind of support!

Thank you and good luck!

– *Sandra*

Would You Like to Know More?

To check what are The 101 Tips That Burn Belly Fat Daily go to my page here:

=> http://projecteasylife.com/101tips <=

To see what are The 7 (Quick & Easy) Cooking Tricks To Banish Your Boring Diet go to my website here:

=> http://projecteasylife.com/7-tricks <=

[BONUS]

Preview of My Other Book, Wheat Belly Diet

(…)

Why Use the Wheat Belly Diet for the Best Results?

If you have tried and failed with other diets, perhaps you were not eliminating the right types of foods. Rethinking wheat has helped people to eliminate the harm it causes to your body. Getting rid of belly fat has thus far been a successful goal for people using the Wheat-Belly Diet.

Very few wheat-based foods are actually healthy for you to eat. The wheat used today, which Dr. Davis calls "Frankenwheat", is genetically modified, and it isn't the same wheat that your parents used to eat.

The modification of the wheat plant has allowed it to be thicker and shorter, so that it is more beneficial for farmers, and more resistant to disease. The bad aspect of this wheat is that it is not as nutritionally rich as conventional wheat, and can damage your health.

The glycemic index is higher in today's wheat than it is in sugar. Some candy bars have a healthier glycemic index than a slice of wheat bread. Glutens that are present in larger amounts in today's wheat cause cravings, and that leads to excess belly fat.

Dr. Davis says that you can expect better results from a wheat-free meal plan, because wheat is more than simply a gluten source. "Frankenwheat" affects the mind, by stimulating your appetite and it can cause depression and anxiety, especially for people who are overweight.

Giving up wheat will allow you to lose belly fat, and can also help in other health issues, such as those mentioned above. People are finally beginning to see the negative effects of today's wheat on their health, and those who stay with the Wheat Belly Diet often find benefits that they did not even expect.

(…)

To check out the rest of the book *Wheat Belly Diet*, go to Amazon here: http://bit.ly/wheatbellydiet

Check Out My Other Books

Below you'll find some of my other books that are popular on Amazon and Kindle as well. Simply go to the links below to check them out. Alternatively, you can visit my author page on Amazon to see other work done by me:

Author page: http://bit.ly/SandraWilliams

Gluten Free And Wheat Free Total Health Revolution

Wheat Belly Cookbook – *37 Wheat Free Recipes To Lose The Wheat And Have All-Day Energy* (http://bit.ly/bellycookbook)

Gluten Free – *The Gluten Free Diet For Beginners Guide, What Is Celiac Disease, How To Eat Healthier And Have More Energy* (http://bit.ly/glutenfreebook)

Gluten Free Cookbook – *30 Healthy And Easy Gluten Free Recipes For Beginners, Gluten Free Diet Plan For A Healthy Lifestyle* (http://bit.ly/gfreecookbook)

How To REALLY Set And Achieve Goals

Goals – *Setting And Achieving S.M.A.R.T. Goals, How To Stay Motivated And Get Everything You Want From Your Life Faster* (http://bit.ly/getsmartgoals)

Prevent And Reverse Diabetes Disease

Diabetes – *Diabetes Prevention And Symptoms Reversing* (http://bit.ly/diabetesguide)

Diabetic Cookbook – *30 Diabetes Diet Recipes For Diabetic Living, Control Low Sugar And Reverse Diabetes Naturally* (http://bit.ly/diabetic-cookbook)

Get Healthy, Have More Energy And Live Longer With Natural Paleo And Mediterranean Foods

Paleo Cookbook – 30 Healthy And Easy Paleo Diet Recipes For Beginners, Start Eating Healthy And Get More Energy With Practical Paleo Approach (http://bit.ly/tastypaleo)

Mediterranean Diet – Easy Guide To Healthy Life With Mediterranean Cuisine, Fast And Natural Weight Loss For Beginners (http://bit.ly/mediterraneanbook)

Mediterranean Diet Cookbook – 30 Healthy And Easy Mediterranean Diet Recipes For Beginners (http://bit.ly/mediterracookbook)

Extremely Fast Weight Loss With Low Carb Approach

Ketogenic Diet – Easy Keto Diet Guide For Healthy Life And Fast Weight Loss, Heal Yourself And Get More Energy With Low Carb Diet (http://bit.ly/ketodietbook)

Atkins Cookbook – 30 Quick And Easy Atkins Diet Recipes For Beginners, Plan Your Low Carb Days With The New Atkins Diet Book (http://bit.ly/atkinscookbook)

Amazing Weight Loss Tips, Tricks And Motivation

Weight Loss – 30 Tips On How To Lose Weight Fast Without Pills Or Surgery, Weight Loss Motivation And Fat Burning Strategies (http://bit.ly/weightlosstipsbook)

Ultimate Guide To Diets – *Choose The Best Diet For Your Body, Live Healthy And Happy Life Without Supplements And Pills* (http://bit.ly/dietsbook)

The Obesity Cure – *How To Lose Weight Fast And Overcome Obesity Forever* (http://bit.ly/obesitybook)

Unique Beauty Tips Every Woman Should Know

Younger Next Month – *Anti-Aging Guide For Women* (http://bit.ly/beyoungerbook)

Hair Care And Hair Growth Solutions – *How To Regrow Your Hair Faster, Hair Loss Treatment And Hair Growth Remedies* (http://bit.ly/haircarebook)

Improve State Of Mind, Defeat Bad Feelings And Be Happy!

Anxiety Workbook – *Free Cure For Anxiety Disorder And Depression Symptoms, Panic Attacks And Social Anxiety Relief Without Medication And Pills* (http://bit.ly/anxietybook)

The Depression Cure – *Depression Self Help Workbook, Cure And Free Yourself From Depression Naturally And For Life* (http://bit.ly/depressioncurebook)

If the links do not work, for whatever reason, you can simply search for the titles on the Amazon website to find them. Best regards!

CPSIA information can be obtained
at www.ICGtesting.com
Printed in the USA
LVOW13s1744230418
574527LV00040B/1770/P

9 781508 791065